AF811689

Brain Foods

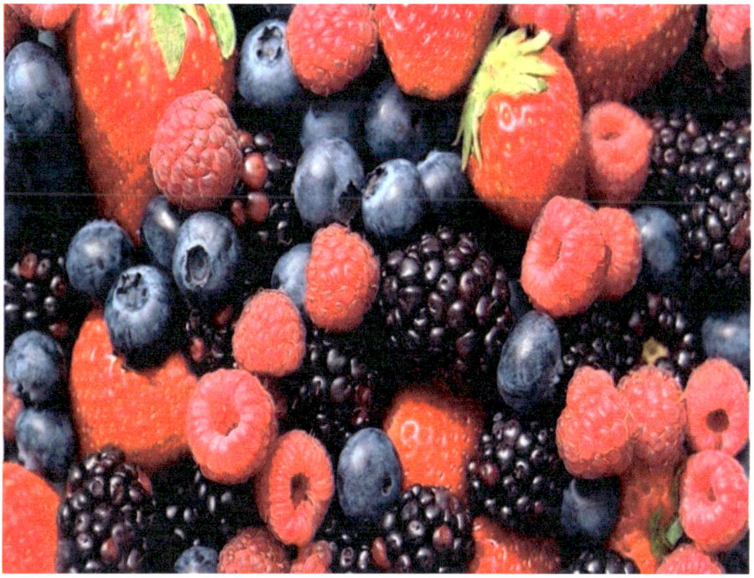

By

Hope Roberts

ISBN: 978-1-7336135-6-9

Published by
Eagles Word Christian Publisher
New York

Printed in the United Kingdom

Dedication

This book is dedicated to

my Mum

Shirley Gale.

The Brain

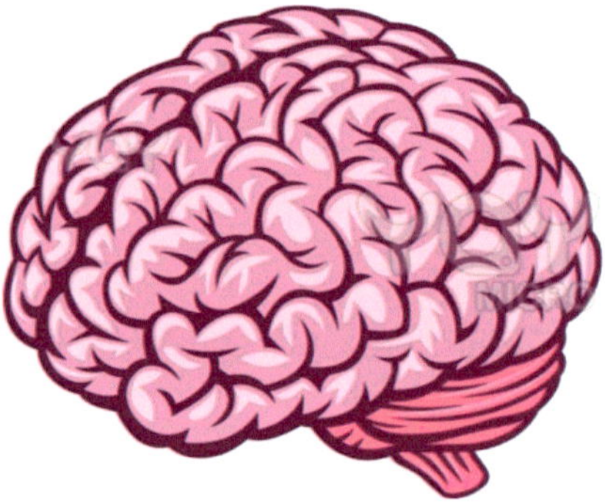

This book is about foods that help the brain to function at a very high level and keep it active and healthy.

Introduction

The human brain is only 2 per cent of the total body weight, yet it needs about 20 per cent of total caloric intake in order to function correctly.

Brain foods are like fuel to the brain. They enhance your health as well as ensuring proper brain function throughout your entire life. According to research, these foods change the expression of the genes in the brain and increase brain communication by creating new brain cells.

Brain foods are the key to protecting people from dementia, Alzheimer's, and other types of brain disease. These foods also help to increase short-term memory.

Disease of the brain ranges from mild to severe, leaving the person completely dependent upon others for basic needs. Eating brain foods on a daily basis can help you to live and enjoy a long, healthy life.

Daily activity is also essential in keeping the brain active. Some examples of activities are: reading, doing puzzles, painting, and daily walks. Healthy habits, such as drinking a lot of water, can also aid in assisting the brain cells to stay active and in good condition for much longer.

Contents

Apples

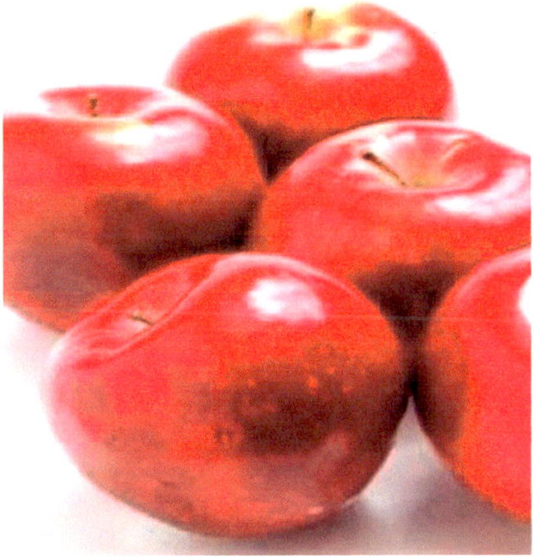

The apple is a fruit rich in vitamins C and B6, zinc, calcium, iron, potassium, phosphorus, and magnesium.

Eating an apple daily, without removing the skin, releases an antioxidant called quercetin. This juice flows to the brain protecting it from free radical damage that can cause memory loss or Alzheimer's disease.

You can eat apples raw, juiced, or stewed.

Serving suggestion: Enjoy a fresh apple every day to complete a healthy lunch.

Avocado Pear

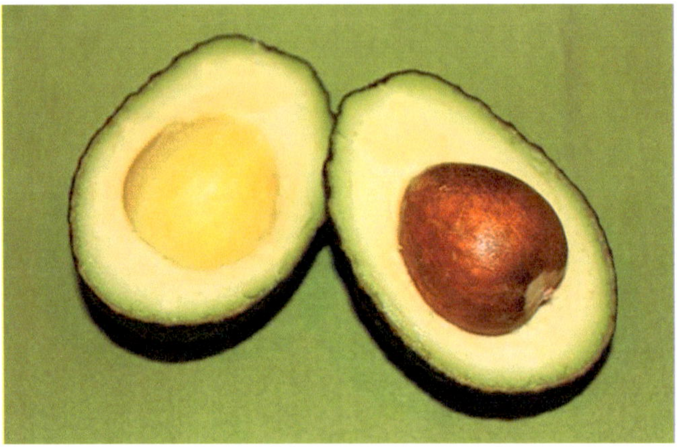

The avocado pear is a tropical fruit rich in vitamins C, E, K, and B6, calcium, iron, potassium, zinc, magnesium, phosphorus, and omega-3 fatty acids.

The fatty acids in avocado pear are beneficial, as they promote blood flow to the brain, keeping the brain function healthy and at its peak. Avocado pear can be eaten in salads or as a fruit or juiced with honey.

Serving suggestion: Enjoy avocado pear with a tuna salad.

Blueberries

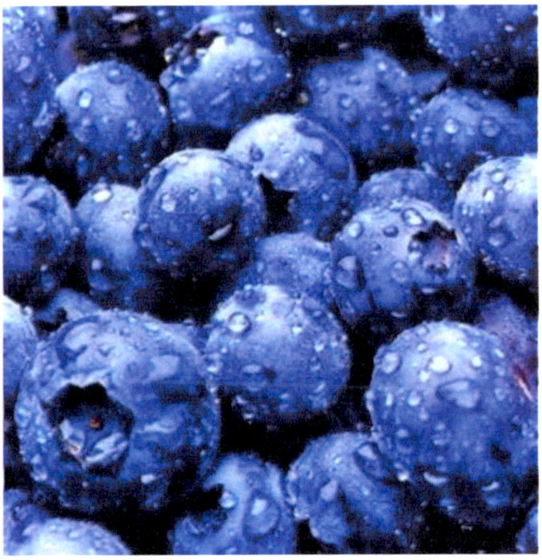

Blueberries are super fruits! Rich in antioxidants, selenium, vitamins such as A, C, E, and B-complex, sodium, potassium, copper, magnesium, phosphorus, and other agents which help to prevent and heal neurotic disorders by ceasing the degeneration and death of the neuron brain cells.

Making blueberries part of a daily meal can prevent serious brain diseases such as dementia and memory loss, along with maintaining sharpness of the brain.

Blueberries can be eaten in porridge, salads, and cereals.

Serving suggestion: Eat a handful of blueberries with your breakfast, lunch, or as a snack.

Grapes

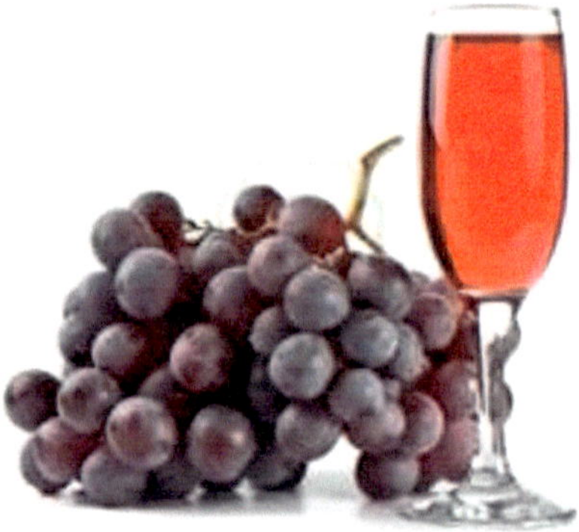

Grapes are cluster fruits rich in essential vitamins and minerals such as vitamins C, B6, and B12, calcium, iron, zinc, sodium, potassium, selenium, magnesium, manganese, and phosphorus.

Grapes can be eaten raw, made into wine, raisins, jellies and jams, or juiced.

Drinking grape juice and eating grapes enhance brain cell function and reduce the risk of developing Alzheimer's disease.

Serving suggestion: Eat grapes as one of your daily fruits.

Pumpkin Seeds

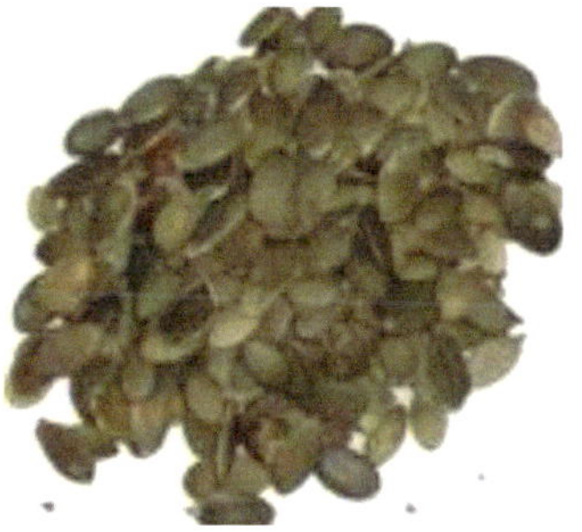

Pumpkin seeds come from a squash (fruit) rich in vitamins E and C, copper, zinc, magnesium, potassium, and other nutrients.

Studies have shown that adding a daily spoonful of pumpkin seeds to food enhances the memory; and the zinc and omega-3 fatty acids both have calming and protective effects on the brain, which help it to function at higher levels, reducing the risk of any brain disease.

You can eat pumpkin seeds raw in your foods and salads.

Serving suggestion: Add pumpkin seeds to your meals.

Raisins

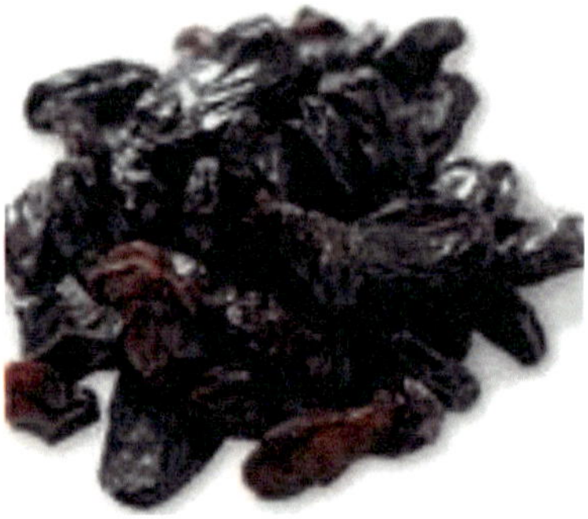

Raisins are dried grapes; they are rich in vitamins C, K, and B6, folate, niacin, iron, folic acid, calcium, and magnesium. These are essential nutrients for the brain.

Raisins are also rich in a very high amount of boron - a powerful brain booster mineral. Boron enhances concentration and memory, protecting the brain from Alzheimer's disease.

Raisins can be eaten in porridge, cereal, and salads.

Serving suggestion: Enjoy a handful of raisins for a delicious snack.

Tomatoes

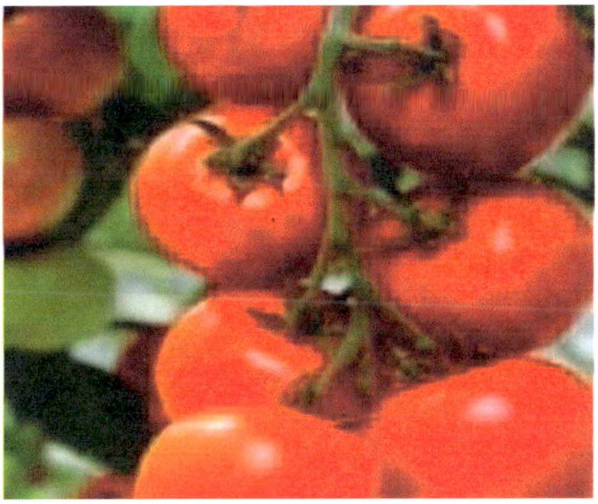

Tomatoes are savoury fruits rich in vitamins, A, C, and K, potassium, iron, calcium, and other minerals.

Tomatoes are also rich in a powerful antioxidant called lycopene which protects the brain cells against free radicals that can cause dementia or Alzheimer's disease.

Tomatoes can be eaten raw, in salads, juiced, or cooked in foods.

Serving suggestion: Drink tomato juice for breakfast.

Broccoli

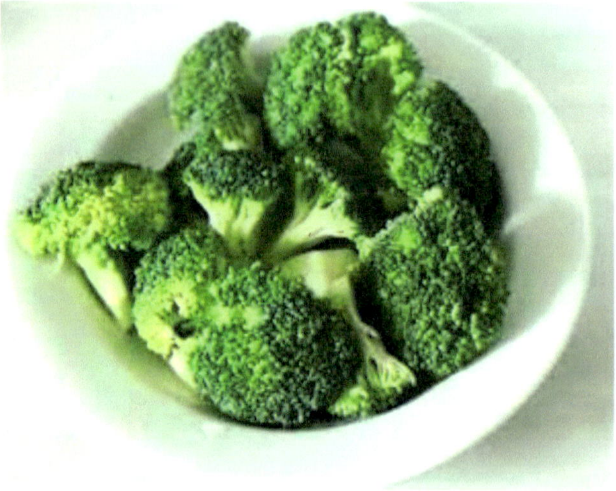

Broccoli is a leafy vegetable rich in many vitamins and minerals such as vitamins A, C, E, B1, and B3, lutein, calcium, iron, zinc, magnesium, phosphorus, and potassium.

Research has shown that a special compound called sulforaphane in broccoli ceases the deterioration of brain cells, keeping them healthy.

Broccoli can be eaten raw in salads or served in soups.

Serving suggestion: Try a delicious juiced broccoli smoothie for breakfast.

Carrots

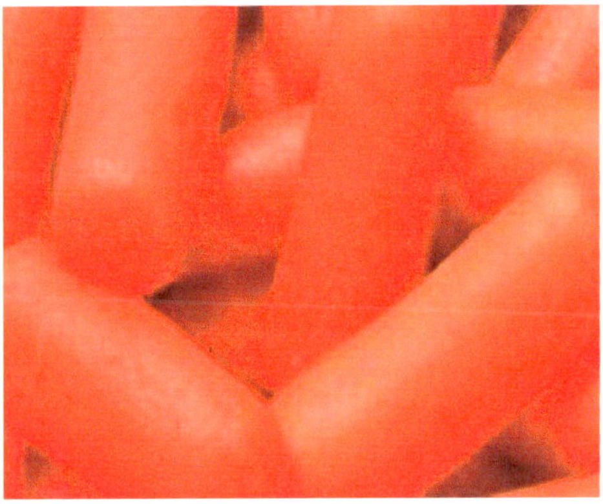

Carrots are root vegetables containing many vitamins and minerals such as folic acid, potassium, magnesium, calcium vitamins A, C, and B6, and many others.

This vegetable is also rich in a compound called luteolin, which helps to reduce inflammation from the brain cells, protecting it from memory loss and dementia.

Carrots can be eaten raw, steamed, cooked, or juiced.

Serving suggestion: Grate a raw carrot and sprinkle it into your salad as a tasty treat.

Spinach

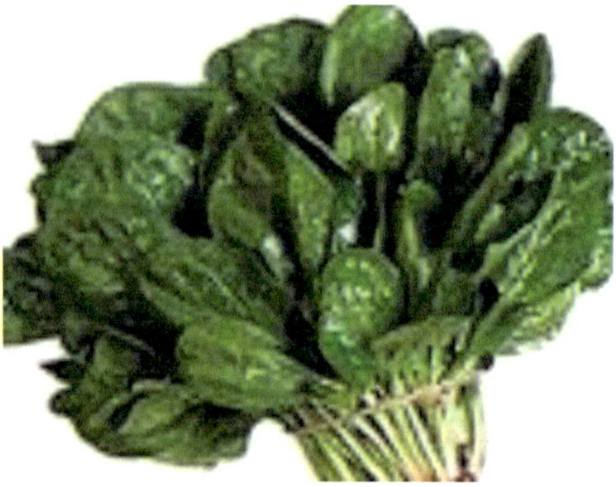

Spinach is a dark green, leafy vegetable rich in vitamins A, C, E, and K, calcium, iron/folate, lutein, and other minerals.

Studies and research have shown that a diet rich in spinach protects the brain cells from free radical damage, helping to reduce the decline of brain cell functions that cause dementia.

Spinach can be eaten raw in salads, stewed, steamed, cooked in soups, or juiced.

Serving suggestion: Like broccoli, spinach can be juiced with other vegetables to make a tasty and delicious smoothie.

Dark Chocolate

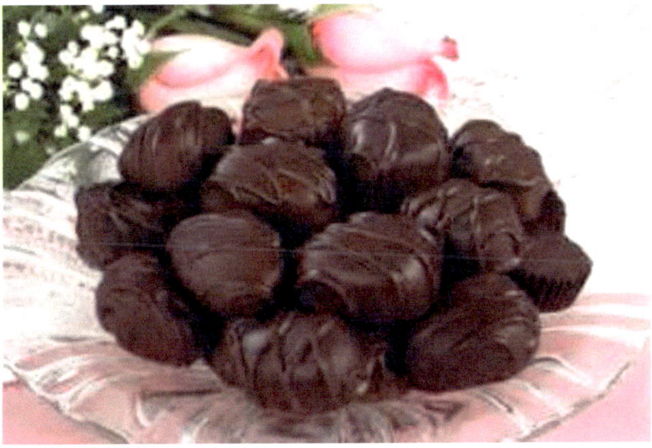

Dark chocolate contains little or no milk. It is rich in vitamins and minerals such as potassium, copper, iron, and magnesium.

Dark chocolate is the key ingredient in boosting blood flow to key places in the brain, enhancing its function.

Rich in antioxidants, dark chocolate helps to keep free radicals from damaging brain cells.

Serving suggestion: Enjoy dark chocolate as a healthy, delicious snack.

Eggs

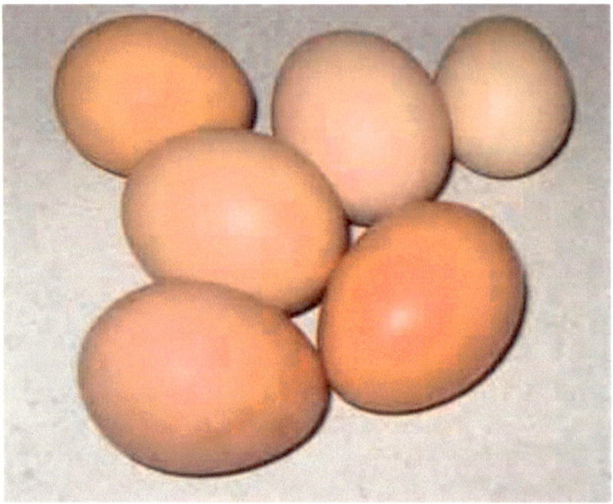

Chicken eggs are rich in vitamins A, B6, and B12, zinc, potassium, magnesium, choline, calcium, and iron. Egg yolk contains choline, which is the key ingredient responsible for good communication among nerve cells which protect the brain.

Research has shown that vitamins B12 and B6 in eggs help to improve memory.

Eggs can be boiled, poached, pickled, scrambled, or eaten raw.

Serving suggestion: Enjoy a boiled egg for breakfast.

Green Tea

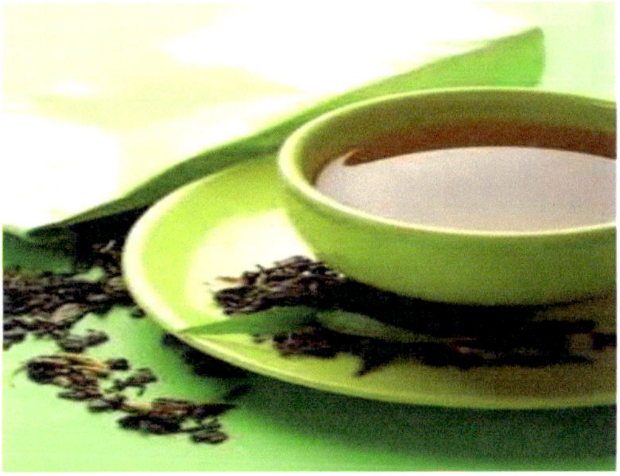

Green tea is derived from a tea plant in Asia and is rich in vitamins, minerals, and polyphenols.

Used as a beverage and for medicinal purposes in Asia, research has shown that the compound polyphenol in tea protects brain cells, keeping them active and healthy.

Green tea maintains a flow of glucose to brain cells, helping them to work smoothly and on a higher level. This protects the brain from dementia and other brain disease.

Green tea can be enjoyed hot or cold.

Serving suggestion: Enjoy a delicious, cooling glass of iced green tea in the summer.

Oatmeal Porridge

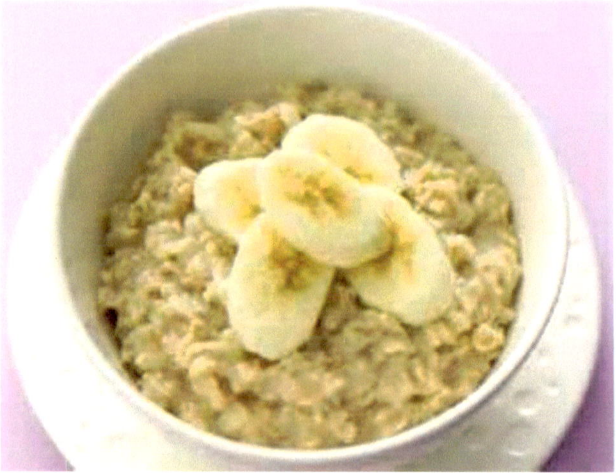

Oatmeal porridge is rich in vitamins B and E, potassium, zinc, and beta-glucan fibre. These nutritious properties give extra energy to the brain and help it to function at healthy levels.

Eating this favourite breakfast porridge daily can be a life-saver.

Oats can be eaten as porridge or made into biscuits.

Serving suggestion: Enjoy oatmeal porridge with a banana, blueberries, or raisins.

Peanut Butter

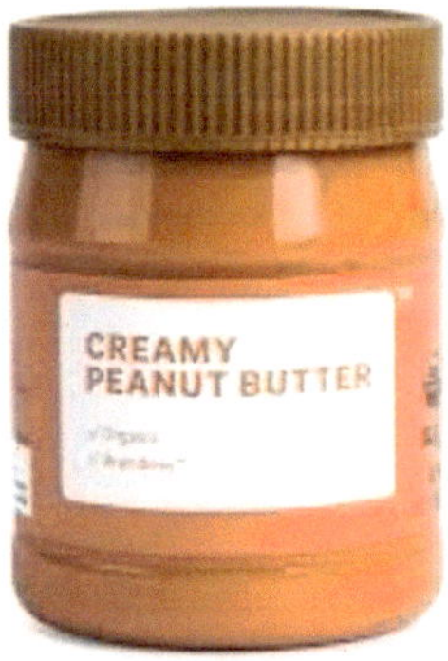

Peanut butter is an herb rich in vitamins A, C, and E, iron, zinc, potassium, copper, magnesium, and many other antioxidants.

A natural brain food, peanut butter nourishes the brain and the nervous system.

The thiamine found in peanut butter converts glucose into energy. Research shows that the brain needs a lot of glucose to keep it active.

Peanut butter is delicious on a sandwich or in stew.

Serving suggestion: Enjoy peanut butter on ice cream as a topping.

Please be aware that people with an allergy to nuts should not eat peanut butter as it can cause severe breathing problems.

Salmon

Salmon contains many nutrients and is rich in vitamins D, B3, B6, and B12, tryptophan, protein, niacin, calcium, magnesium, omega-3 fatty acids, selenium, and phosphorous.

Recent studies have found that the omega-3 fatty acids in salmon help to improve brain function, preventing brain diseases such as Alzheimer's and dementia in addition to improving listening and response functions.

Salmon can be enjoyed grilled, poached, baked, steamed, or stewed.

Serving suggestion: Bake well-seasoned in the oven for a healthy meal.

Walnuts

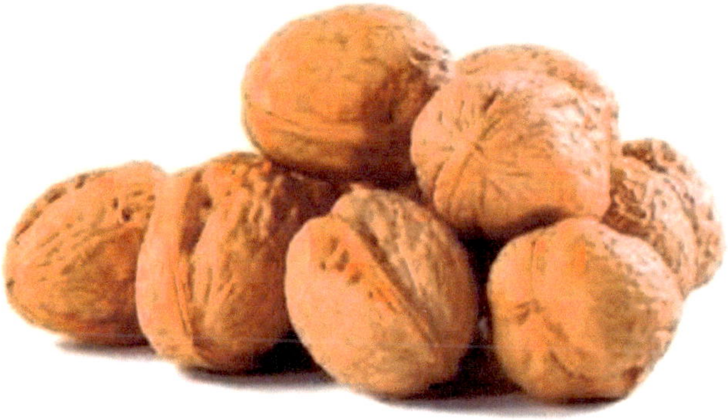

Walnuts are stone fruits rich in vitamins A, C, D, E, and K, beta-carotene, iron, calcium, magnesium, manganese, phosphorus, potassium, sodium, zinc, folate, lutein zeaxanthin, and omega-3 fatty acids.

The essential omega-3 fatty acids help the brain cells to communicate with each other on the right levels, keeping the brain cells healthy and protected. The walnut is also rich in a hormone called melatonin which facilitates sleep.

Enjoy a spoonful of walnuts in cereal, lunch, or dinner.

Serving suggestion: Eat a walnut snack before going to bed as an aid to sleep.

Please be aware that people with an allergy to nuts should not eat walnuts as that can cause severe breathing problems.

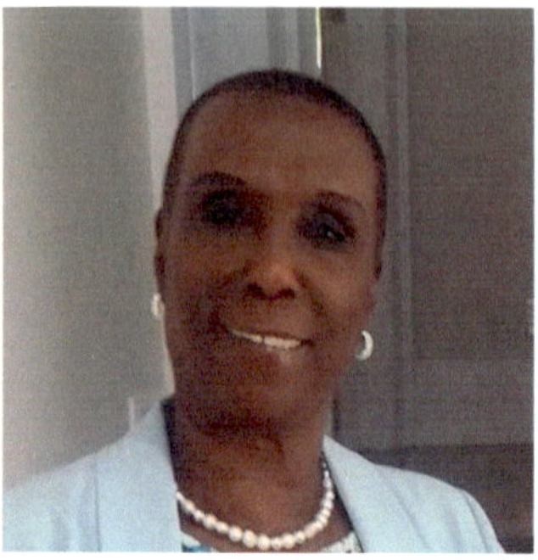

Hope Roberts was born in Guyana, South America. She now resides in England and wears many hats. In addition to her current day job of helping people as a nurse, she is also a poet, writer, and encourager.

Hope began writing in 1986 and has since had her work published in several books and magazines.

She has read and shared her work in schools, and on radio and television.

Made in the USA
Monee, IL
05 November 2026

67945041R00017